FACE YOUR FUTURE

By Verne Weisberg, MD

VERNE WEISBERG, MD

TABLE OF CONTENTS

INTRODUCTION - VANITY IS A MYTH

People get plastic surgery for many different reasons. The most obvious, or at least the one that people think of initially, is out of vanity. This is actually not true; vanity is a myth. The major reason people get plastic surgery is to restore their self-confidence.

A young woman in her 20s had given birth to two beautiful children. She and her husband were still totally in love, but she could no longer bear for her husband to see her naked, because of her stretch marks, sagging breasts and sagging tummy skin. She came to see me seeking surgery to restore the appearance of her breasts and tummy, so that she could once again feel sexy with her husband. Like she, many people won't even take their clothes off at all, or even wear revealing clothing if there's even the slightest possibility that someone else might see. For many young women, oftentimes, there is a lack of much breast development, or sometimes even a significant asymmetry, with one breast enlarging significantly and the other barely developing at all. These situations are extremely embarrassing for the young woman in question and have real impact on her sense of self and wholeness. For these people, plastic surgery is utilized to restore balance in their lives and confidence, which will ultimately lead to success further along in life.

Plastic surgery can restore self-confidence or instill the self-confidence that a person never had because of the way she or he looked, and the way people treated them as a result. As sad as it is to contemplate that people can be mean and nasty just because of they way you look, it's a harsh reality that has existed for as long as humans have been human. We'd like to think that this is a reflection of our cultural values, and to a certain extent that's probably true, but in truth, humans have always been judgmental, and we've always treated people differently based on either the way they look, how tall they are, what color their skin is, how they smell, and even how they sound. While questions such as these can sometimes be addressed with outward improvements such as plastic surgery, obviously the correction of the innate driving forces is beyond the scope of this volume.

A successful C-suite gentleman sought consultation to soften his wrinkles and tighten the sagging neck and eyebrows in order to combat the signs of aging and remain competitive in the marketplace. This may sound odd to you, but you see, as we age, we tend to develop the appearance of an older person despite still having a sense of vitality, fun and energy. Our outward appearance detracts from the perception of our inward energy, and so when we look in the mirror, it becomes upsetting to us because the way we look is not congruent with the way we feel. Older individuals may seek plastic surgery to align our outward appearance with our inward selves. This motivation to have plastic surgery relates primarily to the face, but even other areas of the body, as we age, tend to show the signs of aging and sagging.

For many men, a similar effect to that experienced by women occurs when they have gynecomastia, more commonly known as "man boobs". Many men are self-conscious about their bellies, but this doesn't tend to bother men as much as it does women. Gynecomastia affects especially the younger men, who don't feel comfortable taking their shirts off when they're at the beach. A successful, fit and handsome young father came to see me because he wanted to be able to participate with his children at the beach or at the pool. His children consistently asked him, "Daddy, why won't you take shirt off and come into the water with us." His joy the next summer after having his surgery was beyond what he could express. This was truly life changing for him and for his role as a father. In fact, the changes after this type of plastic surgery really affect every aspect of the individuals' lives and give them back their self-confidence or give it to people that have never had it before in ways that are far reaching.

And what about children? It starts as early as kindergarten, when a small child may be picked on ridiculed for having what used to be referred to as "Dumbo ears". Their ears stick out and people comment on it, and they wind up growing up feeling restricted about the appearance of their ears, trying to cover them up with either long hair or hats. Similarly, while most small children don't have large or crooked noses, as they start to age and come into adolescence, these genetic tendencies start to show up, and they then become either ridiculed for the appearance of their nose or find themselves extremely uncomfortable if someone is taking a sidelong picture of them. For some people, even the fact that their nose widens as they smile is an issue. A girl who grew up with my daughters was often made fun of because of her large, masculine-looking nose. The summer before her senior year of high school, she came to me to have her nose made more feminine. When she had her senior picture done, her parents sent me a copy, with thanks for how the surgery had allowed their daughter to blossom into the beautiful, confident young woman they had always known she was, but others couldn't see before.

And of course, we cannot forget the need for plastic surgery after deforming surgeries, traumas, or birth defects. These are the impetuses for plastic surgery that pretty much everyone gets behind, and no one ever gives anybody a hard time about. Situations such as requiring reconstruction after mastectomy for breast cancer are clearly important and no one ever questions this. Similarly, when someone has a terrible scar from previous traumas or surgeries, everyone agrees that it's reasonable to have these scars made to look as good as they possibly can. Frequently, removal of these scars, especially those of trauma, can have a very healing effect to the psyche, as it takes away the consistent reminder of the trauma that caused it. When I was the Chief of Plastic Surgery at the West Haven VA Hospital, there was a Vietnam veteran who asked for removal of the tattoos on his arms, because looking at them gave him flashbacks to when he was a POW. Even the resulting surgical scars on his arms were welcomed, and his therapy was able to progress.

So, you can see that there are as many reasons for which people seek Plastic Surgery as there are people. So let's look more closely at how to find the best Plastic Surgery for you!

FOREWORD

J im and Barbara (not their real names!) came to see me in my office several years ago. Their last child had left the home, and they were "free". They had an exciting plan for their newfound time together. Travel, adventure, lots of beaches, and hikes were all worked out. They felt young and energized, but when they caught themselves in a mirror or a store window, they were wondering who those two old people were. They didn't like the disconnect between how they appeared and how they felt. They didn't want people on their trips looking at them and treating them like some-one's grandparents, or thinking they couldn't keep up. And they liked being with a younger crowd – loved new ideas, and stimulating conversation. So they decided that their looks could use some sprucing up so that they could look as young and vibrant as they felt. Their goal was to seen as the "Embarassingly Passionate" couple they were in truth.

Over the course of my 28 years as a plastic surgeon, I have had the privilege of serving over 20,000 patients, and

I believe that so many problems can be avoided if people take care and know the right questions to ask, so that they are able to find the right surgeon. The American Society of Plastic Surgeons reports that in 2014, over 12 billion dollars were spent on cosmetic procedures, with over 4 million procedures performed just in the Mountain/Pacific area alone. We are all aware of the numerous celebrities who have had plastic surgery, and that list is actually too long to write. For most of them, things turned out well, however for a notable number of notables, there have been some very public disasters. So much so that right now, one of the most popular reality TV Shows is *Botched,* in which people who have had "bad" plastic surgery show up to a few different plastic surgeons to have the deformities corrected. While this has certainly stimulated public attention, much like watching a disaster unfold on the news, it is disturbing in its significance.

Getting the BEST possible Plastic Surgery is more than just finding the best surgeon. You need a team that works together to support you as well as the surgeon, so that the atmosphere is one of comfort and assurance, and so that the surgeon is in what I like to call a "beautiful state" while operating. There's no room for tension and aggression in the office, let alone in the OR. The old caricature of the irascible surgeon barking orders is one that should be relegated to the trash heap of history.

I believe that the biggest barriers to having success in Plastic Surgery relate to poor research on the part of the person seeking it, poor training, technical ability or even ethics on the part of the Plastic Surgeon, and of course the reality that no mater how carefully and well things are done, we are human beings, and despite everything's having been done correctly, things can and sometimes do go wrong and there may be complications. The goal of any medical process, and certainly any surgery, is to minimize those possibilities.

My desire for this book is to serve you as your "best friend"; to support you in your journey, or in helping people you know with theirs. We will go through the various types of Plastic Surgery that are currently available. We will look at how to evaluate whether this is something that is right for you; how to find the resources to be able to ask the best questions, so that you will be able to get the best Plastic Surgery and Plastic Surgeon for you and therefore the best possible results. I want you to be the person whose life has been changed forever for the better, whose confidence and passion has returned because of Plastic Surgery.

Chapter 1

WHAT'S THE BEST AGE TO GET PLASTIC SURGERY?

A teacher in her mid-forties came to see me one day because her students would always ask her why she looked so angry all the time. She had developed deep furrows between her eyebrows and looked like she had a permanent scowl! But she was the happiest, most cheerful person I'd ever met! Her appearance really had a large negative impact on her ability to connect with her students.

The best age to have Plastic Surgery really depends on what the procedures are and what the side issues may be. There is no set rule for when one should have plastic surgery, certainly, as an adult. For children, it depends on the area. By the time a child is 8 years old, their ear is 80% the size that it will be when they are an adult. Similarly, the nasal bones don't change much from about the age of 12, so having the nose corrected by the age of 16 is absolutely appropriate.

When it comes to the breasts, our judgment has to be very considered, because development in young women may take longer and in some women, it could even take until age 20 for full development. Nowadays, due to the hormones in the foods we eat and the types of foods that we eat, such as those containing sugars that add to the fat in the subcutaneous layer of the skin, breast development tends to start a lot earlier than it ever has before in human history.

Many young women want to have breast enhancement but wonder if it's okay to do it before they have children or whether they should wait. Similar questions are asked about tummy tucks, as well. And older people have started to be concerned about when it is they should consider having any sort of facial rejuvenative surgery such as, eyelid work, facelifts, neck lifts, etc. This is really decided on an individual basis, and can start as early as late 30s or early 40s and may be appropriate in the mid-to-late 70s. It really depends on what type of results one's looking to achieve and what types of health or structural issues have to be dealt with in order to have safe and effective surgery.

I tend to counsel people to have facial rejuvenative surgery when the issues actually start to bother them. Either they notice it in photographs, or as they look in the mirror, or perhaps somebody has commented on it. Some people like to wait until things get further out of hand, and others want to be really proactive and may even start the quest to maintain a youthful appearance in their 20s, with wrinkle blockers such as Botox and even fillers to maintain structural support. It is better and easier to make small changes and corrections early on than to wait until problems get large, obvious and less correctible.

When it comes down to timing, often the questions asked are in reference to school, work, time off, and even summer time or other activities. It's important to be able to plan far in advance so that you can take these issues into account and have the least amount of interference with your normal or desired activities. Frequently, for adolescents, vacation times are the most popular question. As we start to go through the various types of plastic surgery, I will address the issues that need to be considered in order for you to be able to get the best possible results, but first, let's think about how it is that we find the best possible surgeon for you.

Chapter 2

How Can I Find the Best Plastic Surgeon?

F inding the best Plastic Surgeon for you has many facets. It's important first to understand what goes into the training of a Plastic Surgeon and the significance of Board certification and other credentials, because it's important for you to check credentials. Plastic Surgeons all start their professional lives at Medical School. The road to becoming a Plastic Surgeon may take many turns.

My own story began, perhaps, on my first day at Medical School. I had been working in upstate New York as a jewelry repairman, working in gold and silver. I had been a watchmaker's apprentice when I was 16, and had worked after school while in high school repairing jewelry in Manhattan. I decided to go to Medical School later in my college career. I thought I wanted to be a Psychotherapist. And my psychiatrist cousin had recommended becoming an MD over becoming a PhD. So I applied to Medical School believing I would become a Psychiatrist. Talking with fellow first-year students during our first week, we shared why we decided to become doctors and what field we thought we might go into. It was at that moment that I first stated that I wanted to become a surgeon who helped to restore people who had been injured. I didn't really know anything about Plastic Surgery at all. And I pretty much filed that thought in the recesses of my mind as I dove into my studies in basic sciences. I learned anatomy, biochemistry, neuroscience and microbiology in that first year. But the faculty determined that it would be important for us to have some exposure to patients early on (a radical departure from the tradition at that time!). A small group was therefore chosen to learn "normal physical examination". I did not get picked (it was random). But then they announced that there would also be a pilot program teaching normal obstetrical exams, to learn about normal pregnancy and the health of the mother and baby. I was chosen for this.

I very excitedly donned my white jacket and stethoscope and followed the Chief Resident around. And then one evening, as we were making rounds, a call came from the OR that he was needed for a C-section. He brought me along, and I learned how to scrub in and experienced my first surgery. It was a combination of excitement, awe and terror for me. Excitement to be in the OR and learn that I wore a size 7 ½ glove. And terror when I was handed the suction cannula and told to suction the blood. I had no idea how much there would be. As I stood there (nearly passing out!), I thought to myself, "there is no way in hell that I will ever be able to do something like this. What were you thinking"? But then the awe of a baby emerging from the womb struck me like a thunderbolt. I had never witnessed such a thing. I don't even remember how they closed her abdomen, but mother and baby did well. I was late for my date, but I didn't care. Something about surgery grabbed me, and I was hooked.

When summer came, I needed to work, so I did work-study at the Brooklyn VA Hospital in the Neurology clinic. In those days, the Neurosurgeon would come and grab the Neurology residents if they were available to help. But often they weren't, so he tagged me and my classmate Mike to assist him. In brain surgery! I'm pretty sure this sort of thing no longer happens. While I was in the OR, between cases, I wandered around and stumbled upon the Plastic Surgery Chief Resident, Dr. Greg Rauscher. He was already a fully-trained General Surgeon, and was doing surgeries at the VA. He invited me to observe one case. Then he invited me to scrub on the next case. I guess he thought I was serious, because as we were scrubbing on the third case, he said, "this surgery is so easy, *you* could do it. In fact you're going to do it!" Talk about nervous! But I did exactly what he told me to do and the surgery (which was actually very simple) went perfectly. I was hooked. I knew I had to become a Plastic Surgeon. To this day, Dr. Rauscher is a dear friend. I committed to learning how to suture and tie knots in my spare time using a plastic practicing device. I volunteered at the woefully understaffed Pediatric ER at Kings County Hospital many evenings, closing lacerations on children applying the Plastic Surgical techniques I learned. The nurses and the parents were very appreciative. I couldn't wait to go there, pretty much every weekend.

While I had some continued thoughts about Psychiatry, my experience with acutely psychotic women on the locked ward of Kings County Hospital sealed my decision to not pursue a career in Psychiatry. I focused on Plastic Surgery (with a brief thought of Pediatric Surgery). I was able to start my career a year early due to a now-defunct program that my school and Kings County had, whereby you could do your final year in Medical School as your internship year in General Surgery. The day after I graduated with my MD, I had to go back to my duties on the ward, while my classmates took off for the last free summers of their careers. After another year of General Surgery, I realized I didn't want to do five years of it, so I took one of the alternative paths to Plastic Surgery by joining a three-year training program in Otolaryngology/Head and Neck Surgery at Mt. Sinai Hospital. After finishing the program, I had the privilege to be accepted to the Plastic Surgery residency I had wanted to go to since my fourth year of Medical School: Yale University.

Medical School is a tough cauldron that works to select out the best of the best. It's important to remember the startling statistic that even at the best medical schools in the world, 50% of the class is in the lower half! Having said that, that doesn't necessarily mean lower quality. As the prospective surgeon progresses through medical school, their interest in surgery starts to develop and they wind up deciding on what their training will be. Plastic Surgery training programs are extremely competitive. The entry to Plastic Surgery used to be based on finishing a complete residency in General Surgery, Otolaryngology (ENT) or Orthopedic Surgery (in other words, a five-year program before starting Plastic Surgery). Nowadays, most of the Plastic Surgery programs are called "integrated". They begin with Internship, and carefully craft the Resident Surgeon's journey to become a well-rounded Plastic Surgeon.

The decision to be a Plastic Surgeon is made for various reasons, and the Plastic Surgery programs are very discerning in whom they take. Becoming a Plastic Surgeon requires that you are in fact the best of the best. Fortunately, at the point that you are chosen to be Plastic Surgeon, and as you go through your training, your skills are developed and you're judged on those skills, so that when you've finished, you have demonstrated competency in being able to have good judgment as well as good technical skills. Obviously, however, since we are all human, not everyone has the same level of judgment and/or skill. And on top of that is the ability to communicate and bond in an empathetic way with other people, specifically patients. When someone has graduated from a high-quality Plastic Surgery program, it's a good indicator that they know what they are doing, have demonstrated technical competence (in other words, they can actually perform the surgeries) and have been able to communicate well with the staff, their mentors, and most importantly, their patients.

Surgeons have different areas of interest and focus within the field of Plastic Surgery, however. Rarely is a Plastic Surgeon good at everything. Some Plastic Surgeons love to do reconstructive work and micro-vascular surgery, because of their desire to restore. And while restoration is the driving force behind every Plastic Surgeon, some Plastic Surgeons find that their true calling is in employing their aesthetic sense - in other words, the artistic aspect of Plastic Surgery. Making things look as good as they possibly can. This actually requires a strong base in reconstructive surgery to start with, and the best cosmetic surgeons are also skilled at reconstructive surgery. In fact, this is one of the most important aspects of being a good cosmetic surgeon, because, as I mentioned earlier, not everything always goes well, and it's important to have a surgeon who knows how to take care of complications. And any surgeon who tells you that they've never had a complication is lying. As with so many things in life, when everything goes well, things are simple. The true test is how things go when it's complicated and when problems arise. You want to be sure that you are in the best hands.

A singularly important decision point for choosing a Plastic Surgeon is, of course, Board Certification in Plastic

Surgery, certified by the American Board of Plastic Surgeons. Plastic Surgery Societies have wrestled with the question of how they can be certain, or at least assure the public, of the competency of their membership, and have tried very hard to assess this through Board Certification, which is a rigorous process that requires clinical demonstration of competence as well as knowledge. Additionally, you're aided if your surgeon is a member in good standing of The American Society for Aesthetic Plastic Surgery (ASAPS). To become a member of the ASAPS, one needs to have performed a specific minimum number of cosmetic surgeries during the course of each year, and therefore have been able to demonstrate competence and specialty in this area. You can check your surgeon's status by going online at www.surgery.org.

What About Other Types of Plastic Surgeons?

There are Plastic Surgeons who specialize only in the face/head and neck, and those doctors are usually trained in otolaryngology (ENT). As with Plastic Surgeons in general, not all otolaryngologists are comfortable with, or even want to do, Cosmetic Surgery of the face. Those who do tend to specialize, and actually do fellowship training after their general Otolaryngology training. These doctors are known as Facial Plastic Surgeons, and go through similarly rigorous training and credentialing before they are able to obtain these important credentials. If you are considering facial surgery from a Facial Plastic Surgeon, be sure that they have Boards in Otolaryngology, certified by the American Board of Otolaryngology/Head and Neck Surgery, and preferably that they have had a fellowship and are a member of the American Academy of Facial Plastic Surgery.

There are also certain Ophthalmologists (eye doctors) who have taken fellowship training for OculoPlastic Surgery, which is Plastic Surgery restricted to the area around the eyes, specifically eyelids or forehead. After such a fellowship, these surgeons are generally very well trained and qualified as well. They too have to go through a rigorous complete training in ophthalmology (eye surgery), and obviously have had to demonstrate technical as well as academic skills in this area.

How Do I Know Who's the Best For Me?

The way to determine who's "the best" is to speak to former patients, look at testimonials that have been posted for the specific positions you are considering and, obviously, check the public record to be sure that the surgeon hasn't been involved in law suits or had sanctions placed against them by the medical board. Oftentimes, referrals from your own doctor are helpful as well. Once you have decided that you have narrowed down the field, it's time to get on the phone and make appointments to interview the doctors and see how comfortable they are with treating what bothers you, and how you feel in their presence. If you have any doubts in the back of your mind, then you very seriously need to consider if this is the surgeon for you. It doesn't necessarily mean that the surgeon is not a great surgeon, but if you are not able to communicate well, or you don't feel that the surgeon is able to listen to you, then that's probably not going to be a good relationship. Again, when everything goes great, you don't need to have that much of a relationship, but if things don't go great, you need to have somebody that you can trust and feel good about their advice.

Is Every Cosmetic Surgeon Able to Do Every Operation Well?

In fact, not every surgeon trained in cosmetic surgery is comfortable with every operation. Some surgeons love to do rhinoplasty ("nose jobs"), while others hate it. Some surgeons love doing breast surgeries, while others are uncomfortable with it and would prefer to do something else. And some surgeons are particularly skilled at face lifting, or particularly talented at tummy tucks or liposuction. It's good to find out what the surgeon feels best about and enjoys doing, because they tend to do best the thing that they enjoy the most. Don't we all? That said, why don't we get specific? Let's look at each area one by one, shall we?

23

Do I Have to Go to a Big City or University?

While most aspiring Aesthetic Plastic Surgeons want to be "where the action is" – places like Beverly Hills, Miami, Dallas or New York, the truth is that those places are super saturated. It's hard to make any inroads there no matter how good you are. So you can find great Aesthetic Plastic Surgeons in most cities around the world. There are no "secrets" to Plastic Surgery. Gone are the days of a Surgeon's jealously guarding his new technique or insight. We share openly and often. Nor is Aesthetic Plastic Surgery restricted to the ultra-wealthy or the celebrities. It's for literally anyone with the reasons to have it. The key is to look for the training, experience, testimonials and results. And to be absolutely certain you are on the same communication wavelength with the surgeon. The surgeon in the less-congested area is likely to have far more experience than those in the larger cities, because in those densely-populated areas of high competition among surgeons, the experience tends to be diluted – they just don't have the opportunities those of us in smaller communities have. So, don't feel like you have to travel. And it's much more comfortable to recover and do your follow ups near home!

Chapter 3

FACELIFT

Joy was so excited that her daughter's wedding was coming. She got very caught up in the planning process, looking for just the right venue with her daughter, helping her pick out the wedding dress, and as is the case so often nowadays, her daughter was documenting all of this with "selfies". As they were enjoying themselves that evening looking at the selfies posted on Facebook, Joy was mortified to see herself. She thought she was looking at her own mother! "When did this happen?" she asked herself. She realized that almost everyone she knew and loved would be at the wedding, and that the photographs that would be taken would be a permanent record of that day. She had been so excited and had felt so young, free and full of joy, but looking at her pictures, that wasn't the person that she saw. She had to bring her external appearance into alignment with who she was inside. She realized it was time to see the Plastic Surgeon her friends were talking about.

While Joy sat with the plastic surgeon, he explained to her the aging process. She came to understand that as time passed, her skin became thinner, with less elastic tissue, and that her collagen was damaged from years of environmental exposure and internal degradation due to oxidized sugars in her diet. She had never really considered that all of those years eating her low-fat diet, and even a time when she had been a vegetarian, could've had such a damaging effect on her skin. After all, she always used the best products she could buy.

He also explained how, as we age, we lose overall volume in our faces, and that this volume needs to be restored in addition to tightening the support tissues that have become stretched. She wondered how that was accomplished, and he explained how modern facelifts work to restore the appearance of youth, and the soft sensuous curves associated with youth, by injecting the patient's own fat and stem cells into those important areas. She liked the idea that the stem cells contained in the grafted fat could improve the quality of her skin as well as restore the fullness of contours of her younger face. As they looked at old pictures of her he had asked her to bring in, she realized that his plan was sound. The doctor explained that the old style of face lifting, of just pulling and tightening, is what has given strange appearances to many well-known celebrities. Pulling without restoring the volume will only make a tighter-looking old person. His goal for her, he explained, was to return her appearance to where it had been 10 or 15 years ago.

"Well, then, couldn't I just refill the areas that have lost their volume?" she asked. "Do you really have to also tighten and remove excess skin?"

The Surgeon explained that volume alone wasn't usually enough. The supporting structures, especially those that tighten up the neck, needed to be lifted. He further explained to her about the SMAS layer of fascia that would be addressed in the facelift. "Sometimes, we dissect and elevate the entire SMAS structure and secure it upwards. In many people, however, we may only "reef in" the fascia and tighten it up."

Joy had wondered whether she might just need only a neck lift, but she now understood that the loose skin in her neck had actually slidden down from her cheeks, and so this needed to be corrected as well with a face and neck lift. "For some people," the surgeon said, "the aging process hasn't advanced as much, and they may benefit with just a neck lift alone." She realized that she wasn't one of those people.

As they looked at her pictures on the TouchMD screen, she saw how much the skin of her upper eyelids was sagging, and in fact she had often noticed that her eyelids felt heavy. The surgeon explained to her that she had sagging of the eyebrows as well as some extra eyelid skin, and so, to correct this, again a combination of volume (fat) and surgical elevation (Brow and Upper Lid) would be used.

"I have to tell you," she said, "the thought of doing eyelid surgery and a brow lift is a little scary to me." He nodded and told her, "Well, I prefer to use a limited incision for the forehead, to get maximum changes, and combine with fat grafting. And the upper eyelid skin 'sliver' removal is something we usually do under local anesthetic with total comfort. This combination really gives a profound rejuvenating effect." After she had been able to ask all of her questions and have them answered in a way that she understood, they came to a decision about how they would obtain her best outcome. The surgery went beautifully, and the changes were exactly what she had been looking for. She looked radiant at the wedding, and her husband was even more attentive than ever!

Questions to Ask Your Surgeon – What Do Yo Need To Know?

Be certain to ask your surgeon about how confident he or she is that they can obtain the results you seek. And really think about what success will look like to you. It's so important for you to be able to communicate this picture to the surgeon, so that you are both aligned. Ask how often he/she performs this type of surgery. And look at some before-and-after photos. This may be more difficult in facial surgery than in body surgery, since people often don't feel comfortable having their faces out there for everyone to see. It's also good to find out where exactly the incisions and scars will be, since they will be permanent. Most surgeons place the incision just inside the tragus, the little cap in front of the ear canal. But some find it preferable to place it just in front, leaving the delicate tragal skin intact. In men, this is usually the approach, in order to avoid having hair growing where it shouldn't.

You also need to remember that, as with any operation, there are risks of bleeding, fluid collection, numbness. and even visible skin loss. This last one rarely occurs, but when it does, it usually heals well on its own without the need for additional surgeries. Numbness of the cheek skin is the rule, and may take months to resolve, but there could be a permanent numbness just in front of the ear. And be sure that you discuss restoring volume, because this is so important to a natural-looking result. Also ask about drains, which are often used, especially when extensive neck work is done. If you need a drain or two, they are generally comfortable, and easily removed after a couple of days.

Find out about what your post-operative care will be like. Surgeons tend to be very particular about their post-operative care regimen, and it may vary widely between surgeons.

Chapter 4

FAT GRAFTING AND STEM CELLS

I n the early days of liposuction, the obvious question from many women was, "Why can't we take the fat you are sucking out of my tummy and put it into my breasts?" And some surgeons tried this. Unfortunately, you can't just inject a big blob of fat and expect it to live. You see, despite our general cultural distaste for fat, it is a truly remarkable structure. Fat cells store energy in the form of fat (no need to go into the biochemistry here). We are very beautifully designed to be able to withstand long periods of famine. If we hadn't been, we would never have survived as a species. Our basic programing is such that when we find and eat carbohydrates, our body produces insulin, which delivers the carbohydrates to the cells that may need them for energy, and any excess is then brought to the fat cells for long-term storage. Where it sits until our bodies need it and turn on the chemical signals to convert it back into a usable energy source (ketones).

Modern humans are all hard wired the same way (with some minor variations in how this works), to the point that our bodies are always on the defense against starvation. Except that nowadays, we have access to food 24/7, 7 x 365. But we have no way to communicate this to our bodies. We can't just tell our bodies to cease storing. And in an environment with high-circulating insulin, the fat cells cannot release the fat. So many of us are overweight or obese. Those of us who tend to put on more fat and put it on faster likely carry the best genes for survival - they are programmed to be able to survive severe shortages of food. Except that there are no longer such famines (in the Western world).

So, what to do with all that unneeded fat? We already talked about liposuction. But what about using what we remove? Isn't there a way that we can use it? There is!

Fat can be harvested relatively gently with small liposuction cannulas, and prepared in such a way that the debris is removed, leaving just healthy cells and stem cells, which, interestingly, exist in proximity to the fat cells. In fact, since they are denser than fat, when you centrifuge (spin) down the fat, the bottommost layers contain quite a lot of stem cells.

In order for any grafting to be successful, you need to put it into an environment (bed) that is optimal for delivering nutrition to the transplanted cells until the blood vessels grow in, and, of course, you need to have a good blood supply in order to provide these blood vessels. You also have to limit motion and shear forces that could damage delicate, microscopic new blood vessels. So, grafting to a large area requires a painstakingly slow and careful process to ensure that these things are optimized. The idea behind fat grafting (also known as fat transfer or fat transplantation) is to basically cast "seeds" of fat throughout the area you want to enhance.

Now, fat provides volume, but stem cells provide character, if you will. What I mean by that is that the stem cells can adopt the characteristics of the surrounding types of cells that are natural to an area (for example, bone, or muscle, or even nerve tissue). And they can influence the way the fat cells express themselves, as well. Stem cell research is perhaps one of the most exciting fields of the future -- our future! Stem cells can repair or regenerate all types of tissue, and we are starting to see some truly amazing things.

Currently, while neural therapies are being trialed offshore (the FDA highly regulates stem cell research), Plastic Surgeons are successfully using fat grafting to restore contour to the face; but we also noticed that the skin quality improves dramatically, likely due to the effects of the accompanying stem cells. We also use it to correct deformities after surgery, such as in the breast or after liposuction. Dr. Roger Khouri, in Key Biscayne, has truly pioneered the use of large volumes of fat to reconstruct breasts after mastectomy, and other surgeons around the world have shown that fat (and the stem cells that ride along with it) can correct some previously hopeless scarring and pain after radiation. I have had success with this in my own practice.

Unfortunately, the US FDA is proposing legislation that would prohibit the use of fat and stem cell therapy in breast tissue. I don't at all understand their reasoning. This type of government interference can set back extraordinary medical research immeasurably. I hope that we can successfully avoid this.

Chapter 5

THE EYES HAVE IT!

H ave you heard it said that the eyes are the windows to the soul? They are perhaps the most expressive part of our anatomy. Like it or not, the first impression we make depends heavily on our eyes. Eye contact. Softness. Hardness. Anger. Bliss. Which emotions do your eyes communicate?

Most of the people I see in my practice for eyelid issues complain that people are always asking them if they are tired, or if they are sad, or even angry. Of course, they aren't. Nothing could, in fact, be further from the truth. Their facial appearance gives that misleading impression. And how easy is it to convey warmth and love through your eyes if they are camouflaged by folds of skin or dark circles?

In order to understand exactly what you might need to

optimize this area, some anatomy is (of course) required. As usual, I promise to keep it as simple as possible! There is no one structure that "stands alone". The entire upper third of the face works as a unit, and the parts are all intimately connected to each other. The appearance of heavy or sagging eyelids may seem to be just the lids, but more often than not, the forehead and eyebrows have a significant contribution to the effect. Because the skin of the eyelids is the thinnest of our bodies, it is the first to show the signs of aging. There is very little fat between the skin and the underlying muscle of the eyelid, and therefore, the action of the muscles gradually and inevitably causes wrinkles to occur (even in babies - just look at them laugh) that eventually set in. And as the thin layer of fat becomes even thinner, the red color of the underlying muscle may start to show through as dark circles. In our upper eyelids, not only does the skin of the lid thin, but the skin and fat of the eyebrow gradually atrophy as well, and our eyebrow skin starts to sag. This gives us the heaviness of the upper lids, and can even interfere with our peripheral fields of vision - a medically significant condition that is often covered by insurance.

So when I look at the eyes, I need to take it all in. Sometimes, all that's needed is to clean up the crinkly skin so that it is smooth and even (if the eyebrows are OK). And this can be simply and comfortably done, with just local anesthesia ("freezing" the area), with a procedure called blepharoplasty. I prefer to call it "skin sliver". The excess sliver of skin is removed, very fine sutures are placed to close up, and that's it. This can apply to either or both the upper and lower eyelids.

But, is surgery the only option? In the earlier stages, no. Raising the eyebrows ever so slightly with a wrinkle blocker like Botox may be all that's needed. Yes, it's temporary, but it works well in the right person without the need of surgery. And if you start early in your life (20s or 30s), doing this can slow the process of wrinkling in your forehead and around your eyes. For the lower eyelids, oftentimes, all that's needed is a peel, which can tighten the skin. This area can also be improved just by filling the hollow with either your own fat or a very soft, injectable soft tissue filler such as Restylane Silk. The key to doing this is to be very careful and gentle so that there are no noticeable lumps or bumps.

Surgery. "What should I know?" "What are the risks?" "How happy will I be?" "And how much surgery do I need?" The eye area has some very elegant anatomy. Because the eyeball is cushioned in a cone of fat (which gives a shock-absorbing effect as well as allowing for smooth, quick movements), this fat can sag a little and bulge outward, leading to "bags". When we remove the bulging fat with surgery, we need to be extremely meticulous in sealing all of the tiny blood vessels, so that there is no bleeding that could track backwards and put pressure on the optic nerve. Fortunately, this is an extremely rare potential complication, but because its consequences are so serious, your surgeon will always need to inform you of it. Although most people ask to take as much of the skin out as possible, so that things are smooth and tight, the eyelid has no strong support, so if we try to over-tighten, some irreversible problems can occur. What are these?

The key to any great surgical result is to begin with the end in mind. And to know just what you want to do, and, more importantly, are able to accomplish. This vision has to be based on the realities of the individual anatomy. For example, if we were to remove too much skin from the upper lids, you could get a condition known as lagopthalmos, where your eyes may not close completely when you are sleeping, which could result in an irritation of your cornea, or Dry Eye Syndrome (DES).

In the lower eyelids, you could lose the ability of the lid to rise up and contact the eyeball, so that you have a condition known as ectropion (which can also develop on its own when you get very old). This occurs because any excess traction on the lower lid is like putting very heavy drapes on a weak curtain rod -- the center will sag. There may be a need to support the lower lid as part of the surgery, by tightening it up with a suture to the outer corner orbital bone. This is known as canthopexy. Some surgeons will nearly always incorporate this move for all of their older patients. When this is done, the eye may have a slightly upturned appearance for several weeks. And if this is done, the upper eyelid needs to be done at the same time, both for access and to prevent having more hanging of the outer upper lid/ eyebrow skin.

Despite this "traveler's advisory" about eyelid surgery, I find that it is an incredibly fulfilling, safe and comfortable surgery. There is minimal "down time" and high patient satisfaction. But what if the eyelids alone are not the real problem? What if the heaviness is due to the eyebrows?

Chapter 6

EYEBROWS/ FOREHEAD

When I was just starting out in my practice, I attended a lecture by a highly-regarded, creative and aesthetically-attuned surgeon, Dr. Robert Flowers. He was a true artist when it came to the eyes. He practiced in Hawaii (I thought that was incredibly exotic) and while he was the expert in surgery of the Asian eyelid, he was also an expert in all forms of eyelid surgery. Anyhow, at this lecture, he pointed out how important it was to understand and address the forehead - which is part of the eyebrow complex. He showed me how raising the eyebrow (putting it back from whence it came) opened the eyes back up, and restored the appearance of youth. In fact, he stated that the brow lift was actually a young person's operation. He felt strongly that this area was the initiator of facial aging. But in those days, even though Bob was one of the first to appreciate the need to restore volume around the eyes (he invented the "tear trough" implant), we didn't truly appreciate the role of volume for the eyebrows. Plastic Surgeons use the terms Brow Lift and Forehead Lift interchangeably, and I will flit back and forth in this description as well. Brows used to be (and sadly, sometimes are still) seen as needing a strong pull upwards. Which is why people would sometimes look "surprised" after a brow lift (think Kenny Rogers).

So, how can you restore a natural, youthful appearance of the eyebrow area without overdoing it? By restoring volume as well as with judicious elevation. Fat grafting in this area is quickly becoming a hugely important tool. If you look at the eyebrows of young people, there is plumpness in the area under and below the hairs. Back in the 60s, Paul McCartney was swooned over for his "bedroom eyes" because of this fullness and curve. If you look at him today, this is precisely the area that just hangs and makes him look so old. It is therefore important to think three-dimensionally, and restore volume as well as the elevation and suspension of the sagging tissues.

Sometimes volume restoration is all that's needed. This can be done with either your own fat or "large-volume" diluted hyaluronic acid filler (Juvéderm or Restylane), a technique developed by the thoughtful and talented Plastic Surgeon, Dr. Val Lambros. However, it's often not enough, and surgery is needed as well. There are several surgical approaches to the forehead/brow. Traditionally, the Brow Lift was a fairly involved surgery that meant an incision across the top of the scalp, just behind the hairline. This is known as the Coronal Lift. It is still used, but with much less frequency. The advantage was that it is a very powerful tool to raise the forehead and eyebrows. There are several disadvantages as well, which need to be kept in mind. Anytime you make an incision in the hair-bearing scalp, you can lose hair around the incision, which may or may not grow back. Also, with the Coronal incision, there will be disruption of the nerves to the top of the scalp, and you could wind up with an area of numbness on the top of your head permanently. But, there is a very strong elevation with long-lasting results possible using this method.

Endoscopic Brow Lift employs a small surgical telescope ("scope"), so that all of the structures we need to see, protect and release can be visualized through small incisions placed far more discretely in the scalp, thereby limiting any hair loss or nerve damage. While this sounds like the ideal approach, there are some things it may not do as well as the Coronal. Specifically, there may not be as effective an elevation, there may not be as much improvement in the area between the eyebrows (the "11s"), and the elevation may not stay up as well. It is currently the most widely-used approach, and generally produces beautiful results. In someone who has an already high forehead and hairline, this method might cause an undesirable elevation of the hairline and magnification of the forehead length, which could look wrong.

You might wonder if there aren't some less-involved or alternative methods. There are several. The area that sags the most, and therefore contributes the most to the heaviness of the eyebrows, is the Temporal. That's the part of your forehead where you massage when you get a headache. It's one of the first areas that thins in mammals, leading to a hollowing out of the temple and a sag of the tissues down over the lateral (outer) brow. Frequently, this is the most effective area to correct. In some people with subtler sagging, the area can be enhanced/corrected by simply restoring volume. Volume can be subtly restored with synthetic filler, such as Juvéderm or Restylane; some surgeons use Sculptra in this area. "Large-volume" (really only 2 CC per side) dilute Restylane works effectively without causing lumpiness. Your own fat is a wonderful filler, and, as we know, it brings the added benefit of delivering some Stem Cells to the area, which have a rejuvenating effect on the skin.

But, if you have volume loss and significant sagging, then the Temporal Brow Lift can often be combined with volume restoration, using your own fat to not only elevate the lateral eyebrow but fill up the temporal hollow, resulting in a softer, more youthful look. This is an operation that can be done easily under local anesthetic, and doesn't raise the hairline. There will be a thin scar just in front of the hairline, but this is generally well hidden beneath the hair that grows forward and downward in this area.

You and your surgeon will best be able to decide which of these approaches would be best for you.

Chapter 7

NOSE RESHAPING

When I was a Plastic Surgery Chief Resident, I spent a few months in Manhattan on the cosmetic surgery service of the prestigious Manhattan Eye and Ear Hospital. It was December, and since we had a newborn and my wife was a busy Resident as well, I couldn't really move to NYC for my rotation. So, I would get up before the crack of dawn every day and take the train into Manhattan. Sounds pretty crazy now, but what I was exposed to and learned was so exciting that it made it seem perfectly logical. I was fascinated by the parade of teenage girls from Long Island who would come in for the "Christmas Rhinoplasty". The surgeries really made a huge difference in their lives, but it was certainly remarkable just how many people wanted rhinoplasty and got it during that vacation time.

Nose reshaping is known as Rhinoplasty, or, of course, a "nose job", which is the most popular procedure among

13- to 19-year-olds.   Since the nose essentially doesn't change much from puberty on up, it is entirely appropriate to get this surgery as a teenager. The second time in a person's life when the nose becomes an issue and one considers having it reshaped is later in life, when the skin thins on the nose and the nose appears to grow. The old wives' tale that your nose grows as you get older isn't exactly true. What happens is the support of the tissues thins out, and so the skin and the cartilage start to extend and droop.

When you are considering having your nose reshaped, it's most important to ask about the surgeon's comfort with doing the operation, certainly to ask about the surgeon's training, and to ask how many of the operations the surgeon has performed, as well as see the before-and-after photos. As with any operation, it's always important to talk to other people who have had the surgery done if at all possible. It's important to remember that with any facial surgery, there are fewer people who are likely to either allow their photographs to be shown or even talk to people about it. Oftentimes, however, you can talk to a previous patient over the phone, granting them a little anonymity.

What exactly is involved in having your nose reshaped? It really just depends on which areas are a problem. For some people, it's just a minor alteration of the bone, which is curving and giving the appearance of a "hump".   For others, not only does the "hump" need to be removed, the nasal bones need to be more narrow; the tip may need a significant amount of work done so that it looks more refined and delicate. This is the usual scenario, and surgery can be performed either through an endonasal ("closed") approach or an external ("open") approach also known as a "rhinoplasty". A lot of it has to do with how much tip work is done, and when more tip work needs to be done, we have a tendency to do the "technique", so that there is more direct visualization of the cartilages and they can be better manipulated. Otolaryngologists (ENT Facial Plastic Surgeons) have a lot of familiarity with working on the nose from inside the nostrils without outside incisions, and may have a tendency to favor the endonasal approach, though the popularity of the "open" approach has continued to expand as we've trained more and more surgeons with this technique. I think part of the reason that so many have been trained in this way is that it's a lot easier to teach and there tends to be a little greater amount of predictability in the result.

What could go wrong? Well, aside from not getting the appearance you were looking for, there can be asymmetries, curves, twists, and even collapses of some areas due to the "memory" of cartilage. And you can get problems with your airway – in other words, difficulty breathing through your nose. If you have septal work, you could even get a septal perforation! Most of these are unlikely, but the most common are asymmetries or crookedness. And the nose changes as we age (just look at old and recent pictures of Harrison Ford, or even Sting before he had his nose corrected) so asymmetries and crookedness could show up decades later.

Regardless, even in the best of situations, there will be some swelling that will, at first, disguise the refinements you will ultimately see, so please be patient!

And speaking of vacation time, you should plan to take a good week-to-two-weeks where you can hide out a bit. After surgery, you will have bruising, and certainly you will have a splint on the outside of your nose, so you'll be pretty visible. Not that I've never been on airplanes and noticed people with big splints on their nose! I've even seen people on airplanes that have clearly had facelifts! You never know what you are going to find when you board a plane.

Chapter 8

BREAST AUGMENTATION AND RELATED SURGERIES

B reast augmentation is a very popular procedure for women who have gone through puberty, so it sees its peak from ages 20 through 29. That is not to say, of course, that women don't continue to seek breast augmentation well into their later years, because they do. Many factors go into the decision to have breast augmentation, and while lack of development is the most obvious, the major stimulus in seeking this is the loss of volume or sagging that occurs after bearing children or losing weight. Similarly, as women age, the support structures of the breasts loosen and the breasts start to sag. It's of great interest to contemplate that for the majority of women, their feminine identity is intimately entwined with their breasts. I do not presume to understand all of the nuances of the psychology and sociology relating to this, but the importance of breasts to a woman's identity cannot be understated.

Many people feel that it's the men who are pushing the women to enhance their breasts, but this is rarely the case. Certainly, there are instances where people have gotten breast augmentation at the urging of their husbands or lovers. I had a patient who came back to see me about 15 years after her breast augmentation, asking to have her breast implants removed, because she had finally divorced a man that had been fairly abusive to her, and it had been his idea alone that had caused her to get breast augmentation. At the time I originally saw her, she'd professed to have this desire entirely of her own, and it wasn't until several years later that she admitted she had never wanted them herself. Fortunately, this is a pretty rare circumstance, but certainly one about which each individual needs to be clear.

Breast augmentation is an incredibly common procedure, and when done properly, so that the appearance is natural and soft, it restores that sense of femininity and balance that allows a woman's self-confidence to blossom. The impact on self-confidence from breasts that are either small, sagging or both crosses all socioeconomic boundaries. It's remarkable how people who otherwise are incredibly confident and powerful have this area that causes a deep-seated sense of inadequacy in their femininity and power.

The Implant: Saline or Silicone Gel?

When you are considering breast augmentation, there is so much noise on the Internet with regard to how one is supposed to go about it, it becomes difficult to make decisions. The first decision, after deciding that this is something worth pursuing, is what kind of implant to get. The decision between a saline-filled implant versus a silicone-gel-filled implant is a lot simpler than one would think. Unfortunately, back in the early 90s, the FDA came up with a pretty radical sweeping decision to place a moratorium on the use of silicone gel implants. Their decision-making process will probably remain forever a secret, however it's unfortunate that the reaction was based on silicone implants of a design that had long ceased to be manufactured. By this, I'm referring to problems we had with the earliest silicone implants related to the decisions by engineers to make the softest possible implants (because it was felt, erroneously, that the reason breasts felt hard after augmentation was that the implants were too firm). The engineers changed the number of crosslinks in the silicone polymer and made silicone that was virtually liquid with an incredibly thin shell. These shells were very porous, and the oily silicone that was contained within leached out and was then able to be picked up by the body's natural cleaning system, the lymphatic drainage. This resulted in silicone being seen in lymph nodes far away from the breasts themselves, and also didn't cause any improvement in the capsular contracture rate. Capsular contracture is when the natural scar tissue that forms around the pocket containing the implant thickens and tightens. This thickening and tightening squeezes down on the implant, increasing the internal pressure and therefore giving the result of hardening. There are a number of factors that contribute to this; we control for as many of these factors as we understand, and currently our rates, nationally, for capsular contracture are under 4% in general.

What we've learned over the years is that, in fact, the silicone gel needs to more "cohesive"; that is, it needs to be more like a solid, so that even when the gel is outside of the silicone shell that contains it, it doesn't spread or lose its shape to any great extent. The modern silicone-gel-filled implant really hasn't changed since the early 90s (because the FDA hasn't allowed for any additional changes or research) and has proven to be a reliable implant that doesn't leak or leach out. The implants are very durable, and the silicone itself does not appear to present any health risk. The FDA had concerns that there were health risks related to silicone, despite the fact that prior to the breast implant controversy, silicone was actually the gold standard for lack of reactivity by which other new implantable materials had to be measured. I know this has been a bit of a long and convoluted story, but the takeaway is that modern silicone gels are very safe, and certainly, in my opinion, are the best type of implant to place.

The Muscle: Under or Over?

The next decision is whether this implant should be "under" or "above" the muscle. The reason implants were ever placed under a muscle in the first place was related to the high rate of capsular contracture that we noticed from the earliest implants. As I mentioned before, there are a number of reasons for which breasts may develop capsular contracture after augmentation. But 25 or 30 years ago, it was felt that with movement of the implants, the capsules would not tighten. Patients were instructed to constantly massage the implants, to move them around so that there would be a very generous pocket that would supposedly keep them soft. Additionally, it was felt that if the implant were placed under the pectoral muscular action, the muscular action would aid in the movement of the implant and therefore keep the capsule from contracting. We now understand that no amount of movement is going to prevent the capsule from tightening, because we now understand the physiology and anatomy of the capsule and the myofibroblast cells that cause it to tighten. For many years, though, we taught residents to perform breast augmentation only under the muscle, in order to try to decrease capsular contracture and visibility of the implant, so with time, this became almost a dogma.

I personally feel that the admonition to keep the implants under the muscle is one that has occurred merely because we have lost sight of why it has occurred in the first place. If a woman has enough soft tissue coverage (in other words, breast and fat), then the surgeon can easily place the implant over the muscle. (In many women, however, especially those who are very thin, an additional layer of soft tissue coverage may be desirable, and this certainly would be an important reason to place the implants under the muscle.) If you re-search on the Internet, there will also be the suggestion that having the implants under the muscle makes it easier to read a mammogram. This really isn't true, as the muscle is really a very thin layer in most people, and, in fact, when the muscle is over the implant, the muscle winds up thinning out due to the pressure of the implant underneath and the pressure of the tightness of the tissues over it. In most situations, the radiologist won't actually see the muscle and won't be able to reliably predict whether the implant is above or below the muscle. So the reasons to make a decision to go above or below the muscle have little to do with avoiding capsular contracture (the rate is only slightly less for under the mus-cle than above), or even, in many cases, with visibility of the implants. They have mostly to do with how much thickness or padding a person naturally has to cover the implant and make it less visible. Another reason to go under would be to keep the implant from showing wrinkling, though even un-der the muscle, implants (especially saline-filled implants) can still show wrinkling.

A lot of women wonder if the implant over the muscle looks less natural than under, however it's anatomically more natural for the implant to be over the muscle than un-der. Going under the muscle may change the depth and the appearance of the armpit and with flexion of the pectoral muscle, the implants may definitely move around and the breasts look odd. It's a decision that really needs to be made with your surgeon.

Do I Need A Lift?

A common reason to seek breast surgery is to get a lift. So many women ask me to put their breasts back up on their chest the way they were when they were teenagers. Unfortunately, we can't just push the breasts up and attach them to something that would hold them in place. Breast lifting is actually a breast "pushup" procedure that relies upon the already-unreliable soft tissues of the breast to create a pillar and support underneath. This actually works pretty well when one realizes that you are trying to reshape the stretched-out skin envelope to hold up the internal breast tissue. A challenge comes when somebody wants to be lifted *and* enlarged, as these two operations tend to work against each other. The other problem with trying to go too large and lifting is that implants above 400 CC tend to have a fair amount of weight, which encourages sagging long term.

Complications of Breast Augmentation Surgery

Capsular Contracture

The most significant complication that concerns a breast surgeon is that of Capsular Contracture. This is a problem that can be very minor, where the breast just feels a little firm, or it can run the gamut all the way up to the point of being very hard, displaced and round-looking, and even painful. How do you know if you have this condition? It can be heralded by a feeling of tightness or even pain, and the implant may seem to rise up on the chest. Oftentimes, the first indication is a rounding off and visibility of the upper part of the implant on the affected side. One of the concerns with this tightening of the scar tissue is its effect on the implant. It can cause wrinkling, which in turn can lead to loss of structural integrity (i.e., a hole), and so the contents of the implant can be exposed. For saline, this translates to a deflation, and for the new silicone gels, to gel outside of the implant (though contained in the capsule). Wrinkles in the implant shell are the cause of deflation or rupture.

Research has been done to try to isolate the cause of Capsular Contracture and the only sure finding in research has been some underlying, sub-clinical infection or colonization by bacteria. This is a fairly old study, and because of that, the recommendation was made to avoid at all costs the contamination of the pocket and to use an antibiotic irrigation period. This is certainly the standard of care for breast augmentation, and at all times, the pocket is irrigated and the implants are treated with an antibiotic solution. Unfortunately, this doesn't totally prevent the problem. There are often times where this occurs several years after the initial augmentation, and while there are thoughts that this might relate to momentary release of bacteria into the bloodsteam, such as from an infection like sinusitis or dental work, there's no clear association.

Unfortunately, there are aspects of Capsular Contracture that we are probably a long way from fully understanding. One of the areas of concern is something called biofilm. A biofilm is actually a micro-ecosystem in which bacteria can live and be protected from the immune system. While not necessarily causing an actual infection, the presence of these bacteria may trigger the myofibroblast cells in the body to lay down collagen and thicken and tighten the capsule. When Capsular Contracture occurs, the treatment is based on the severity of the condition. For the most mild ones, there is some thought to either use external ultrasound as a modality or just give a course of medicine that interferes with the action of the myofibroblasts in the hope that the breast will soften. Occasionally, this works; however, it hasn't been very consistent.

If a decision is made to do surgery to fix Capsular Contracture, then this surgery will require that the capsule be as completely removed as possible, and the implant will need to be changed as well, since we won't know for certain that there hasn't been some microscopic "sub clinical" colonization (biofilm) of the implant. In general, while many surgeons feel that this is a difficult operation and that there may be removal of normal tissue, very little normal tissue should be bothered at all. Often, these capsules can be easily "shelled out" in their entirety. This is frequently a successful operation, but it doesn't prevent a recurrence. If it comes back a second time, it's worth trying one more operation, but if it returns a third time, probably breast augmentation is something that shouldn't be redone. At the very least, the implants should come out and time should be given for everything to heal before considering trying again. Capsular Contracture is actually easier to treat if the implant is over the muscles, because when the implant is under the muscle, the capsule is tightly adherent to the chest wall and ribs and may be difficult to completely remove.

Other Complications:

Implant Infection. This can show itself as pain, swelling and redness. An infected implant is fortunately very rare. It generally requires, at least, the placement of an irrigating catheter, so that the pocket can be irrigated with an antibiotic solution, in addition to administering antibiotics intravenously. If this is not successful, then the implant must be removed, and not replaced for several months. You would have to consider whether to remove the un-infected implant as well, in the interest of avoiding very obvious asymmetry. This is when it's important to have a great relationship with your surgeon, so that you can work together to come up with the best solution for YOU.

Bleeding and/or Fluid Collections. As with any operation, these are rare but known complications. On the rare occasion that there is bleeding in the post-operative period, you may need to be returned to the OR to have the blood removed and the open blood vessel controlled. Fluid collections are very rare after breast augmentation. If they occur years after the surgery, then we raise a suspicion of ALCL (see below).

Asymmetries. Sometimes, the implants may not settle into the exact position the surgeon desires. In such a case, you have to decide how tolerable this is to you. If you decide to have surgery to correct this (lower or raise the fold), It may be possible to perform this under local anesthetic. There must always be a spare implant on hand in case the surgeon feels the current one needs to be replaced (it can get injured)

Wrinkles. Wrinkling can run the gamut from barely palpable (you can feel it) to always visible, and any variation in between. The thinner you are, the more likely it is you will have to deal with this issue. Saline implants were notorious for wrinkling and scalloping of the implant edges. Replacement with gel-filled implants may provide an easy remedy to the situation. Many people think that wrinkling can be prevented by placement of the implants under the muscle. While the likelihood of visible wrinkling is somewhat less, it is not eliminated. The muscle overlying the implant tends to thin, and if this happens, the edge of the implant and traction wrinkling may become visible even through the muscle!

Numbness. As all of the tissues get stretched, so do the nerves. This can cause a temporary numbness in part of the breast, all of the breast, or just the nipples. Caution to be patient is advised, however, as this usually resolves itself over the course of weeks, though it could take months to get better. More frequently, patients notice hypersensitivity of the nipples for a few weeks afterwards. While permanent numbness is possible, it's fortunately pretty rare.

ALCL. There is an extremely small risk of developing Anaplastic Large-Cell Lymphoma (ALCL). This is a T-cell lymphoma, which appears to have a very localized manifestation. In other words, it doesn't appear to escape the capsule. It presents as a swelling of the implanted breast years after the augmentation surgery. There is no special testing or monitoring for this. The FDA, which seems to be more than happy to do anything it can to regulate breast implants, suggests that the likelihood of developing this is so remote that there is no advisory, and as such, stands behind its recommendation that implants are safe.

Chapter 9

LIPOSUCTION

M y awareness of liposuction arose in the early 1980s, when I was still an ENT Resident. Reflecting back on that time, it's funny to imagine that there could be any controversy. After all, it's now a household word, and has been proven effective millions of times since those early days. But in 1984, it was scandalous if you did it. In fact, you could be excluded from the medical staff, or at least shunned by your peers, for doing something so "out there".

But it caught on quickly, and in 1987, I found myself in a beautiful mansion outside of Toronto, learning from the pioneers in the field. Fresh off my fellowship and being a Professor at Yale, I had not been prepared for what a private clinic would be like. It looked like a gorgeous hotel or even museum. Every detail had been thoughtfully and lovingly executed through the vision and passion of Dr. Lloyd Carlson. The mansion had not only two operating rooms (perhaps even more), but also a true operating theater, where the attendees could sit and observe live surgery going on just down the hall! We were truly treated as if we were in a prestigious University. And in those days, it was easy to have surgeons from around the world come and actually do the surgery live, so we got to see the pioneers operate. And on a rotating basis, we also got to be in the OR to observe firsthand and up close. For highly trained surgeons like myself and those in the audience, this was an enormously useful way to learn. And it allowed myself and other teachers to bring back state-of-the art techniques to our students.

Liposuction was "invented" by the creative French gynecologist, Yves-Gerard Illouz (1929-2015). His patients had frequently asked him whether he couldn't just suck out some fat from their thighs while he was doing a procedure on them. Until that time, fat had only been removed with a sharp, cutting device, which had, to say the least, poor results, often resulting in bleeding and fluid collection, and even uncorrectable scarring and tissue necrosis. This history was what colored the negative inclinations of the medical community when first liposuction was introduced. As Dr. Illouz was contemplating his suction curette (used for routine D&C), he thought, "Why not just try it?" And so, in 1977, liposuction ("Lipolysis") was "discovered". Although the early results were remarkable, there were still limitations due to blood loss and surface irregularities, but being able to remove fat without making a large incision was revolutionary.

When I met Dr. Illouz for the first time at that meeting in Toronto, and had an opportunity to speak with him, I was impressed with his genuine caring and desire to help as many people as possible. He was truly selfless. Confirmation of his character is easily found, as he was a founder of Medecins Sans Frontieres (Doctors Without Borders). I felt that the understanding and practice of liposuction had only just scraped the surface, and I have personally worked since that time to refine the technique, not only in terms of results but also for patient safety and comfort.

Of course, as with everything else, growth does not occur in a straight line. So, what were the lessons and how were they learned? A number of techniques and theories have come and gone over the years, including "superficial" liposuction, whereby the fat was removed primarily from just under the surface of the skin, with the idea that the irritation of the skin would cause it to shrink down through scarring. This led to too many surface irregularities. And it didn't really get the skin to tighten. We have come to understand that by combining small cannulas and dilute anesthetic solutions (tumescent or "super-wet" solutions), we are able to safely remove larger quantities of fat, with much less surface irregularity. There have been some notably harsh lessons, as some surgeons felt emboldened to push the envelope. We learned that too much fat removal could result in fluid shifts that could lead to shock and death (we all recall Kanye West's mother's sad story). And have we learned just how much of the lidocaine in the local anesthetic can be used while still maintaining a large margin of safety.

Today, most surgeons have specific volume restrictions to which they hold themselves, so that patients can achieve their desired outcomes in a controlled, safe manner. While some states have legally regulated the total amount of fat that can be removed, these numbers are arbitrary, and in general are far, far below what is scientifically safe. Nevertheless, liposuction is a tried-and-true standard of care, and is performed regularly by almost every Plastic Surgeon, and, indeed, by other specialties as well.

How Is It Done?

Modern advances in local anesthesia have made liposuction a procedure that can be comfortably and safely performed without the patient having to go to sleep, although that option is always available. By stabilizing the fat with tumescent solution, a more even reduction can be made, and bleeding is generally negligible. Liposuction works by passing a thin steel tube into the area to be treated. This tube has very small holes on one end and is attached to a source of suction on the other end. This "cannula" has a blunt tip, so that there is as little trauma as possible to the tissues. In this way, we are able to minimally damage any blood vessels and nerves that course through the area. And with smaller cannulas, the incisions necessary to introduce the cannula are small as well, and can therefore be placed in such a way that they are generally invisible to the eye.

Liposuction is routinely and safely performed in almost any area of the body. It is most commonly done in the abdomen, hips, thighs, back, face and arms. It is also a technique that has been successfully used to remove some lipomas (benign fatty tumors), although this doesn't generally get all the matter out.

As the fat is removed by passing the cannula back and forth (generally in a rapid manner - many surgeons break a sweat!), the skin will shrink over the reduced volume of fat. The extent to which the skin is able to shrink is the key factor in determining just how much fat can be removed from an area. As we age, the firmness/thickness and overall tightness of our skin decreases, so that the older we get, the less fat can be removed without having to address unsightly skin sagging or wrinkling.

How Can I Be Sure I Am Getting The Best Liposuction?

As is the recurrent theme of this book, the key is in selecting the right surgeon for you. You need to feel comfortable that the surgeon is truly listening to what your desired outcome is, and that previous patients are happy. Before-and-after photos are the baseline, and patient testimonials are even better.

You must have realistic expectations. Liposuction is not a weight loss technique. What's most important to your success is realizing that liposuction works best in localized areas of stubborn fat -- the areas that persist even when you are at your fittest. It is truly a body-shaping surgery. You will not really notice a big difference on the scale. In fact, in the first month or so, you may find that your weight has not changed or even gone up. Relax; this is just from the water accumulation as a result of swelling. The swelling from liposuction doesn't generally resolve until about twelve weeks. And many of my patients have told me that, as good as the results were at three months, they were even better at six months. So don't run out and buy new, smaller clothing just yet. Be patient.

Can The Fat Be Moved Fom One Place To Another?

Well, yes, it can! This is, in fact, the most exciting and growing area of fat surgery: fat grafting. A graft is tissue that is moved from one place to another without its intact blood supply (so it requires a great "reception area", one with good blood supply, and protection from movement while the new blood vessels grow in). Fat grafting is successfully used in facial rejuvenation, correction of contour deformities, breast reconstruction and augmentation (still a bit controversial), as well as the illustrious Brazilian Butt Lift. But I'll describe these to you in detail in a separate chapter!

Chapter 10

ABDOMINOPLASTY (TUMMY TUCK)

A Tummy Tuck is a powerful operation for restoring self-confidence. It can restore the attractive shape to your abdomen. It can take away that "pouch" that has people asking when you are due. The Tummy Tuck is a great operation for people who have extra skin after pregnancy, childbirth or weight loss. You cannot tighten the skin by exercise or by diet. Generally, it needs to be removed. After you've had a Tummy Tuck, you will likely go down a size or two in your clothing and feel good about how you look. You can finally see the results of your hard work once the sagging excess skin is gone. You will be more confident in the Yoga studio, and in the bedroom. Many people tell me that it is a truly life-changing surgery.

When I first started my practice, I performed the abdominoplasty the way I learned it in my residency at Yale. Like most everyone else. With a small twist. The traditional approach is to raise up the abdominal skin at the level of the deep fascia that covers the six-pack muscles (rectus abdominis), after releasing the belly button from the skin so that it stays attached to the abdominal wall, pull down the skin, remove the excess, and bring the belly button out through a new opening in the newly-tightened skin. And we would need to put in at least two silicone rubber drains, because there would always be a collection of fluid afterwards. The drains prevented the fluid from accumulating, so that the skin could heal to the abdominal wall. Drains are not really comfortable, and people would have a lot of discomfort and pain afterwards for a week or two. And sometimes, fluid would continue to accumulate after the drains were removed, which necessitated multiple visits to the office to "tap off" fluid until it stopped. But I thought that if I left a thin layer of fat on the deep fascia, maybe the lymphatic drainage wouldn't be so disrupted and there would be less fluid accumulation. That was my "twist". It was helpful, and reduced the length of time the drains had to be in, but it wasn't enough to allow me to not use them.

Then one year, probably about fifteen years ago, I attended a great conference that is put on every year in Miami and heard a Plastic Surgeon from South America speak about not using drains and how he had modified the technique. This was intriguing, and I got closer, but still couldn't eliminate them - though I got down to one. The following year, there was a presentation by a French surgeon who presented a very logical approach, having analyzed the patterns of lymphatic drainage of the abdominal wall, and I finally learned the trick to being able to reliably perform the operation without any drains, leaving the lymphatic systems as undisrupted as possible, and limiting the extent to which the area was "undermined". In other words, doing just what was necessary, and very carefully, using liposuction to help in thinning the fat layer and to help mobilize the skin to move the way I wanted it to. Combining this with a progressive suturing technique has revolutionized my practice, and I have been fortunate enough to be able to teach this to other Plastic Surgeons who have had similar success.

How Do I Know If I Am a Candidate for a Tummy Tuck?

If you have excess skin in the lower abdomen and thickening in the midsection of your body that wouldn't be corrected by just liposuction alone, you are likely a candidate. If you have lost a lot of weight, or you have carried large children, or had a lot of internal fat that you've released, then you are likely a candidate, and may need to have the fascia that envelops the muscles tightened with sutures. The surgery I use today in my practice is one in which there is generally only mild discomfort (sometimes none), unless the muscles have been tightened. You will need to take it easy for a couple of weeks afterward, though no bed rest.

You should try to move around as much as you can - either walking or when lying down. You want to encourage free flow of blood and lymphatic drainage from the legs.

What Complications Should I Know About?

As with any operation, bleeding, fluid collections and infection are possible. There can be a loss of skin near the incision, and certainly there can be widening or thickening of the scars. Contour irregularities are possible after liposuction anywhere in the body, and this area is no exception. The major concern we have with any abdominal surgery is VTE - Venous Thrombo Embolism. Blood clots can develop in the large veins of the leg or pelvis that can cause swelling of the lower extremity, or even break off and go to the lung (Pulmonary Embolism). This is a complication that is higher in women who smoke and/or use Birth Control pills (but not IntraUterine Devices or IUDs). If it occurs, you may need to be on blood thinners for some time. Fortunately, even though the incidence is higher in this operation, it has been very rare in my practice. But we are always on the lookout!

What If I Don't Have That Much to Get Rid Of?

You are very fit, but you just have a little skin above the pubic area that is unsightly. A full Tummy Tuck may be too much and you may not have enough laxity to get all of the skin out from between the belly button and the pubic area. In this case, you may be a candidate for a "mini" abdomino-plasty. This operation can be supercharged with skin tight-ening using "Injectable" Radio Frequency (ThermiTight). While you can never restore the bounciness and springiness of a teenager's skin, we can often tighten the skin with this technology, which is a great new tool. At your consultation with your Surgeon, if you truly think you are a candidate, ask if this is an option for you.

Chapter 11

ARMS AND OTHER AREAS

As we age and as we lose weight, loose skin can detract from the celebration of our successes. We want to be able to wear a short-sleeve or even sleeveless shirt, but the flapping wrinkled skin is so obvious and embarrassing. Do you wish you could wear shorts, or a bathing suit, or go for a run without the inner thighs chafing? Or do you have a roll below or above the bra strap?

These areas can present a challenge, and the problems show up in predictable ways based on anatomy. Our skin is attached to our support structure (bones and fascia) in very specific places. We have these Zones of Attachment to keep our skin "suit" from sagging down around our ankles! But what happens is that the tissue above these strong attachments loses its thickness or tightness and starts to sag. The Zone of Attachment prevents it from progressing further down, but results in the skin's hanging over this attachment, resulting in either wrinkles or "pouches". This is best illustrated by thinking about the female breast. The reason it has a fold, and can develop the teardrop shape, is because of the tight Zone of Attachment around the chest (the inframammary fold). This is the same attachment that causes the bulge and fold of skin on the back. In the arm, the adhesion zones are designed to prevent sagging of the skin across the elbow and down to the wrists. We don't sag longitudinally from shoulder to wrist; we sag circumferentially from biceps to triceps. This is the cause of the "wings" that can occur when we raise our arms. So, in order to tighten the upper arm skin, we have to think three-dimensionally again. But mostly, we need to reduce the circumferential distance. And this is done either with just liposuction, with liposuction combined with ThermiTight, or with an arm lift, known officially as a Brachioplasty.

How Do I Know Which Operation IS the One For Me?

It mostly depends on the quality of the skin. If you have a lot of fat excess and have skin that is springy enough to contract down over a reduced volume of fat, then liposuction alone (or in combination with ThermiTight) might be the best route for you. If your skin has been stretched out or lost its springiness, then you may need some skin removed, possibly in conjunction with liposuction and/or Thermi-Tight.

What Can I Expect from the Brachioplasty?

You can expect a reduced upper arm circumference. You want to be certain that the scar can be placed farther back, towards the triceps, so that it isn't so obvious when you wear arm-revealing outfits. But even with great placement, the scar may rotate forwards a little as it heals and become a bit more detectable. It's important that you are fully accepting and aware of the possibility of having a visible, thick and/or red scar. But if the scar is pretty hidden in most poses, then you won't really be bothered by it and you will be thrilled with your new shape!

Possible Complications?

As with all surgeries, the usual players - infection, bleeding, fluid collections, and thick or red, or even tender, scars. There is also a potential for areas of numbness. I try to stay away from the areas where the nerves live, so the likelihood of this happening is pretty small. But some surgeons go down to the fascia of the muscle, and then not only are the sensory nerves at risk, but there can be interruption of the lymphatics, which could result in fluid collection for a while. Some surgeons use drains. I would try to avoid that, were I in your place.

What About My Thighs?

The inner thighs are very similar to the upper arms, and the possible complications are pretty much the same. This incision tends to be placed in the groin crease, and travels back to the fold under the butt. It can be uncomfortable during the healing phase, and has a likelihood of migrating downward for a (usually small) distance. In other words, it could become visible. Not in shorts, but perhaps in a bathing suit. Some surgeons use a scar that goes longitudinally on a line from the knee to the apex of the inner thigh. I find that this requires a very careful technique to try to avoid lymphatic collections. And the scars may be particularly noticeable. But in the right candidate, it's exactly what's needed. Unfortunately, while it may look like all you need to do is liposuction, the inner thigh skin doesn't really like to tighten up, so most of the time, liposuction alone would be inadequate. Some skin usually needs to be removed.

And Other Areas?

Skin can be removed from almost anywhere. The tradeoff is always the location and appearance of the resulting scars. Talk to your surgeon carefully so that you fully understand what you might expect from the operation.

Shining Some Light on Cosmetic Lasers and Devices

Eric Dohner, MD

I've asked my dear friend, Dr. Eric Dohner to write this chapter, because of his extensive expertise and passion for lasers. He is the Founder and Director of the New York Skin and Vein Center in Oneonta, NY

What are lasers and How do they work:

LASER stands for **Light Amplification by Stimulated Emission of Radiation**. When the sun shines on us, that light, has many different wavelengths in the light beams, including light we see by, light that warms the earth, and light that causes skin cancer. A laser on the other hand generates light in a single wavelength. Why is this important? Well because rather than seeing things with sunlight that is reflected off of the objects, laser light is absorbed by the "target" to affect and treat very specific structures such as brown spots, blood vessels, skin tissue and hair follicles. All of these structures attract different wavelengths of light which is why only one laser won't treat all skin and medical conditions.

In general, lasers affect a skin structure by heating it up more than the surrounding structures. This is why, for instance, we can treat broken capillaries filled with blood on the face without affecting skin next to it. The lower the wavelength number, the more superficial (closer to the surface) the laser penetrates and vice versa. Thus 532 nm does not get nearly as deep into the skin as does the 1064 nm laser. Medical/cosmetic lasers are usually divided into categories based on the structure they affect.

Vascular and Pigment Lasers

These are lasers with light that is attracted to blood in vessels and the pigment in brown spots. Some are obviously better than others in certain conditions. Currently the world's best vascular laser is considered the Excel V by Cutera. This laser has two wavelengths: "532nm KTP" and "1064 nm Nd Yag". The number refers to the wave-length of the light and the letters refer to the elements involved in forming the wavelength. The 532 KTP is attracted to red blood vessels and to brown pigment. It is amazing for rosacea, broken capillaries, sun spots, freckles, etc. Your doctor needs to be very careful with this laser on darker skin such as Italian or Indian due to it's effects on skin pigment. The 1064 Nd Yag laser however is very safe for darker skin because the light is not very attracted to pigment. It is used for blue or purple vessels and for hair removal.

Another type of vascular laser is the 585/595 nm pulsed dye laser (PDL). This has fallen out of favor by many dermatologists due to its limited use for only vascular problems but it can be very effective for certain conditions such as port wine stains and red scars. The most commonly used PDL is the Vbeam Perfecta by Candela.

The 755 nm Alexandrite laser is effective at treating pigmented spots but not blood vessels. The most common device is the Apogee by Cynosure. Intense pulse light devices (see below) are also effective at vascular and pigmented spots.

Depending on the condition treated, it can take 1 to 6 treatment sessions to see resolution of your problem.

Hair Removal Lasers

These lasers have been developed specifically to heat up and kill hair follicles. If you destroy the hair follicle, then the hair shaft cannot grow. It takes approximately 6 treatments to kill most of the hair follicles because the laser can only kill hair follicles when they are actively growing. Hair is in active growth only 15% of the time. So a single treatment only kills 1/6th of the hair. Unfortunately, various medical conditions can stimulate the growth of hair follicles so even though a person has gone through a course of treatments, she may develop more hair in the future.

The other big factor in hair removal lasers is the color of the hair and the color of the skin. Lasers can only kill hair that is brown or black because the light is attracted to those colors. This means lasers do not work on white, grey, blond or red hair (this is where medical electrolysis works well). Also your skin color is important in deciding which laser is used: the darker the skin, the longer the wavelength needed so that the skin pigment does not absorb the heat.

The 810 nm diode laser is the fastest and most comfortable hair removal laser. It is manufactured by many different companies but the most famous is the LightSheer by Lumenis. The 755 nm Alexandrite laser is also useful for hair removal. The safest wavelength for darker skin is the 1064 nm Nd Yag laser because this wavelength is "color blind" to pigment. This wavelength is generally slower and the most uncomfortable. Intense pulse light devices (see below) are also effective at hair removal but must be used very carefully on anyone with darker skin.

Resurfacing Lasers

These are lasers that actually remove part of the skin which allows new skin to grow. This process smoothens out wrinkles, improves skin texture and color, and tightens skin. This type of procedure has much more "downtime" than other laser treatments: anywhere from 1 to 10 days of recovery. However, the results can be amazing.

Two different laser types are used for resurfacing: the 2940 nm Erbium and the 10,600 nm Carbon Dioxide (CO_2) laser. Both of these laser heat up the water in the skin so they do not target just one specific structure. The difference between the two wavelengths is the depth that they penetrate: the Erbium laser cannot go nearly as deep as the CO_2 laser thus it does not provide as good results usually. In the past these lasers were used to remove the entire top layer of skin and, while the ultimate results could be great, the recovery, healing process and the risks were more than most people would endure. It was then found that the laser beam could be split it into hundreds of tiny beams. This "Fractional CO_2" treatment allows only a fraction of skin to be removed while surrounded by untreated skin. This gives almost as good results with much less recovery time and risk and it has become the gold standard for resurfacing treatments. Recently "non ablative" lasers have been used for skin improvement. These lasers heat up the skin and collagen but don't actually remove any skin. This has much less recovery time and risks but requires multiple treatments to achieve any visible results.

The resurfacing fractional CO2 lasers that are most commonly in use today that give the best results are Deka Smartxide "DOT", Lumenis Ultrapulse and Accupulse, Fraxel Repair, and Cynosure Affirm. Other devices on the market are not true fractional devices and are not thought to give the best results. The Cutera Pearl and Sciton Profractional are erbium lasers with less smoothing and tightening effects.

The skill and experience of the doctor who performs your treatment is as important as the laser used to treat you. Choosing to undergo a resurfacing procedure is a major decision not to be taken lightly. Another important detail prior to a resurfacing treatment is conditioning the skin to get it ready for the resurfacing. This involves using tretinoin (Retin A) or a strong retinol for at least 6 weeks before the the laser treatment to prepare the skin to respond properly.

Tattoo Removal Lasers - Q switched and Picco lasers

532 and 1064 wavelenths

other wavelengths

also help with pigmentation issues like melasma, hemosiderin deposition, Nevus of Ota, etc.

Skin Tightening and Fat Reduction Devices

Radio frequency - Exilis, Vanquish

Ultrasound - Ultera

Laser - Sculpsure

LED light

What does a laser treatment feel like? Most of the lasers feel like a rubber band snap. For the sensitive person we have a very effective numbing cream and a machine that blows cold air onto the treated area. This combo makes the treatments very comfortable.

What does the skin look like after a treatment? The area treated generally looks slightly red like a mild sunburn afterwards. If we need to be very aggressive then you can be more swollen and red. Any brown spots we treat will be slightly darker for a week or so and then flake off.

Adverse effects of laser: Because lasers essentially heat up the areas being treated, sometimes side effects can occur. The most common of these are pain, redness, bruising, blistering and crusting. These are all temporary. Laser treatments can occasionally reactivate herpes infections or cold sores on the lips. If the skin is burned by a laser treatment, then pigment changes can occur especially in dark skinned individuals which may be permanent. The changes in the color of the skin can be darker or lighter including loss of pigment entirely. Scarring is always a possibility but very rare.

Are there alternatives to Lasers for vascular/pigment/hair removal? There is a class of light devices called Intense Pulsed Light (IPL). These are not single wavelength lasers but rather have multiple wavelengths. These were developed as a cheaper alternative to lasers, but they just don't have the efficacy that most lasers do. There are some states like New Jersey that only physicians can operate lasers so IPL's are popular in those states so that the nurses may perform the treatments.

Who can and should operate lasers? You may often read that only board certified dermatologists or plastic surgeons should perform your laser treatments but this is incorrect. Most physicians do not have the time or inclination to run their lasers. Well trained nurses and technicians who are supervised by a well trained physician have the time and interest in performing your treatments. The only exception to this are resurfacing laser treatments which should only be performed by physicians.

CONCLUSION

I hope you've found this work to be of service to you. I am
grateful that you've taken the time to read through it.
The field is evolving more and more quickly. We are at the
dawn of three-dimensional printing of prosthetic limbs, and
of organs. We are just barely scraping the surface of our
understanding of the regenerative capabilities of Stem
Cells.

I know that someday, perhaps not that far off, the types
of surgeries we now think of as state of the art will be relegated to the history books. So many operations and techniques that I learned as a Plastic Surgery Resident at Yale
have gone by the wayside.

I am excited for us to Face Your Future together! It is
indeed a bright one, filled with wonder, love and "Embar-
rassingly Passionate" moments.